Dumbbells

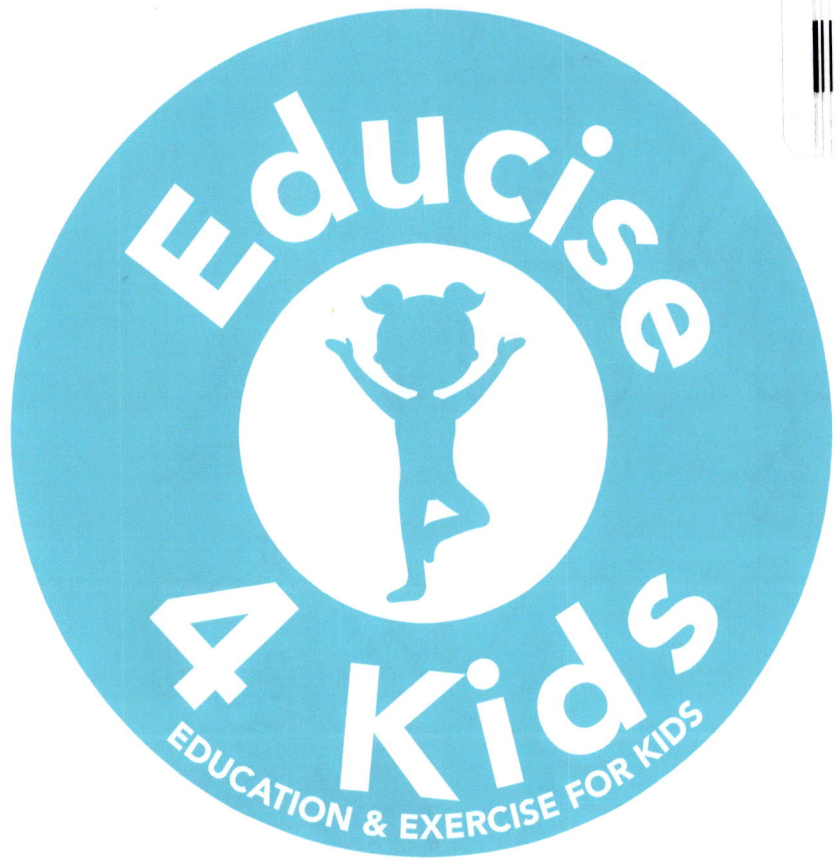

Educise
4 Kids
EDUCATION & EXERCISE FOR KIDS

Created By
Priscilla Fauvette

Illustrated By
Bernard Fauvette

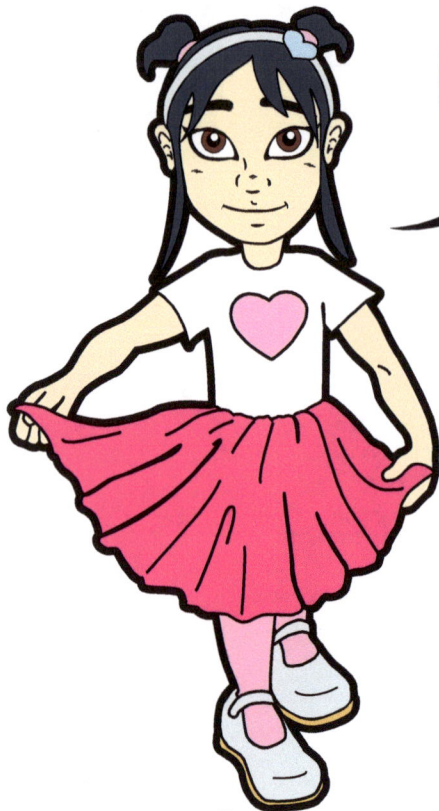

Lin

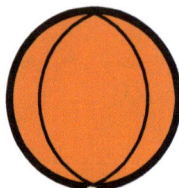

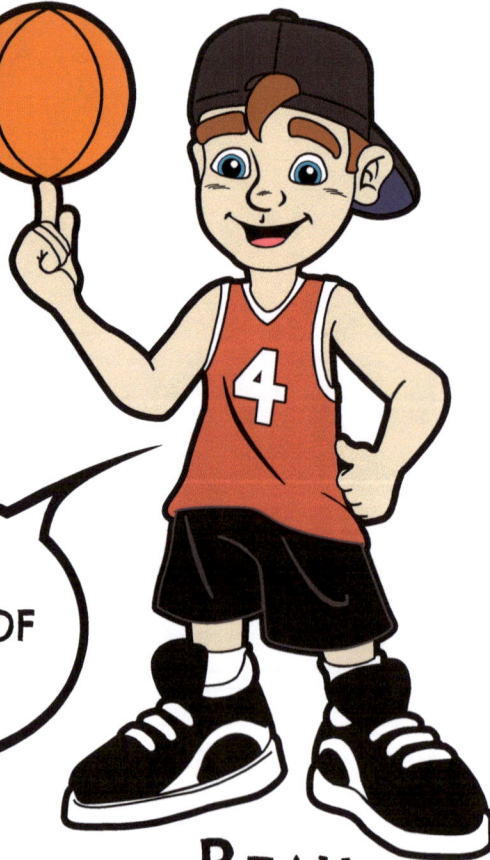

Beau

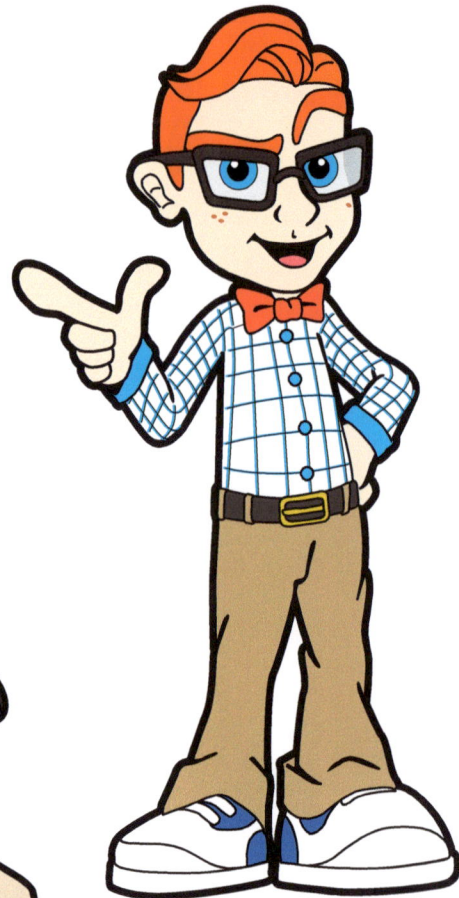

Caden

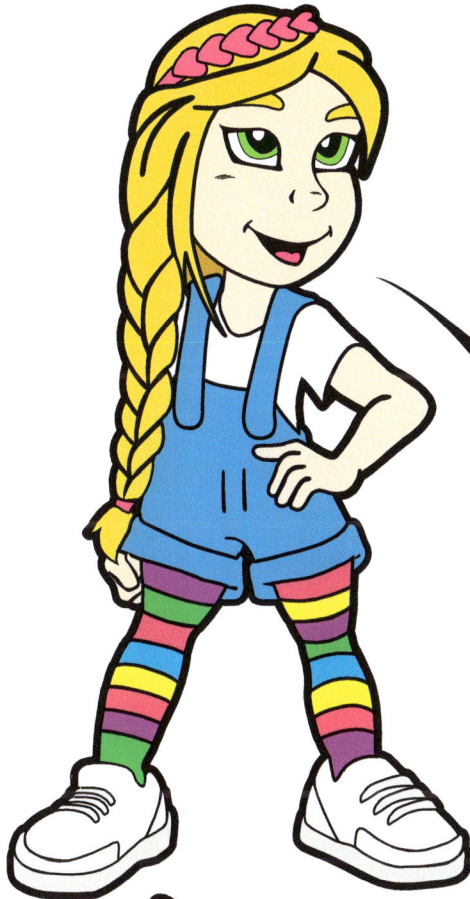

SOPHIE

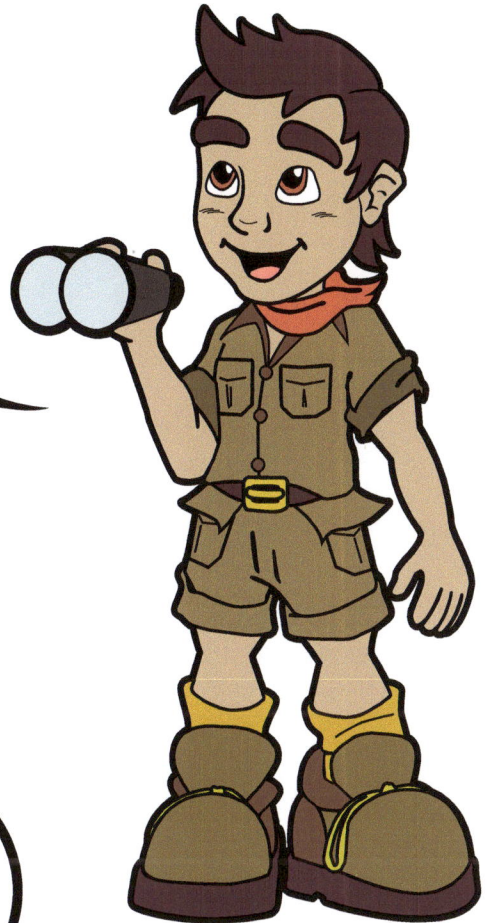

ZAC

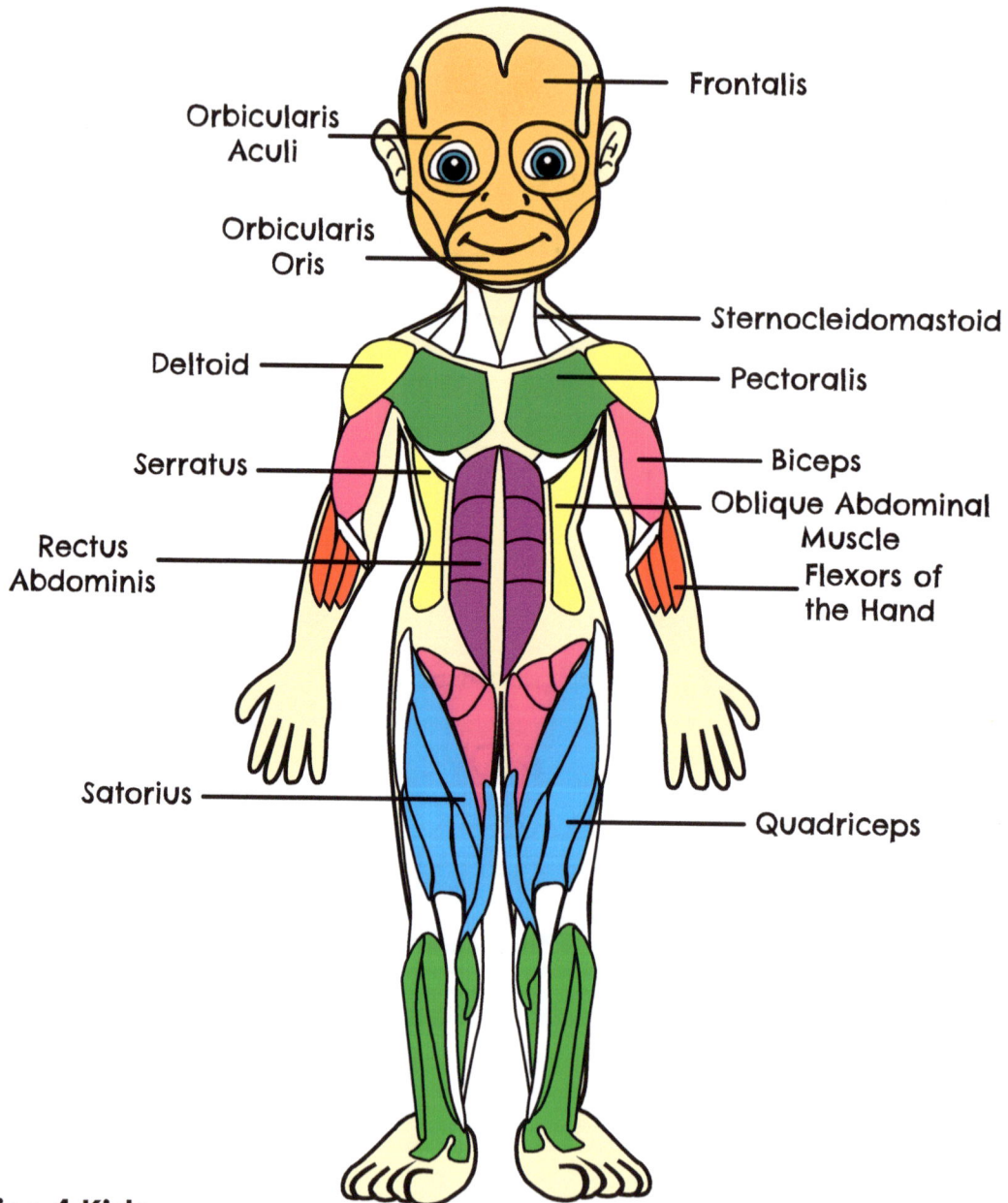

Anatomy

Frontalis

Orbicularis Aculi

Orbicularis Oris

Sternocleidomastoid

Deltoid

Pectoralis

Serratus

Biceps

Oblique Abdominal Muscle

Rectus Abdominis

Flexors of the Hand

Satorius

Quadriceps

Anatomy

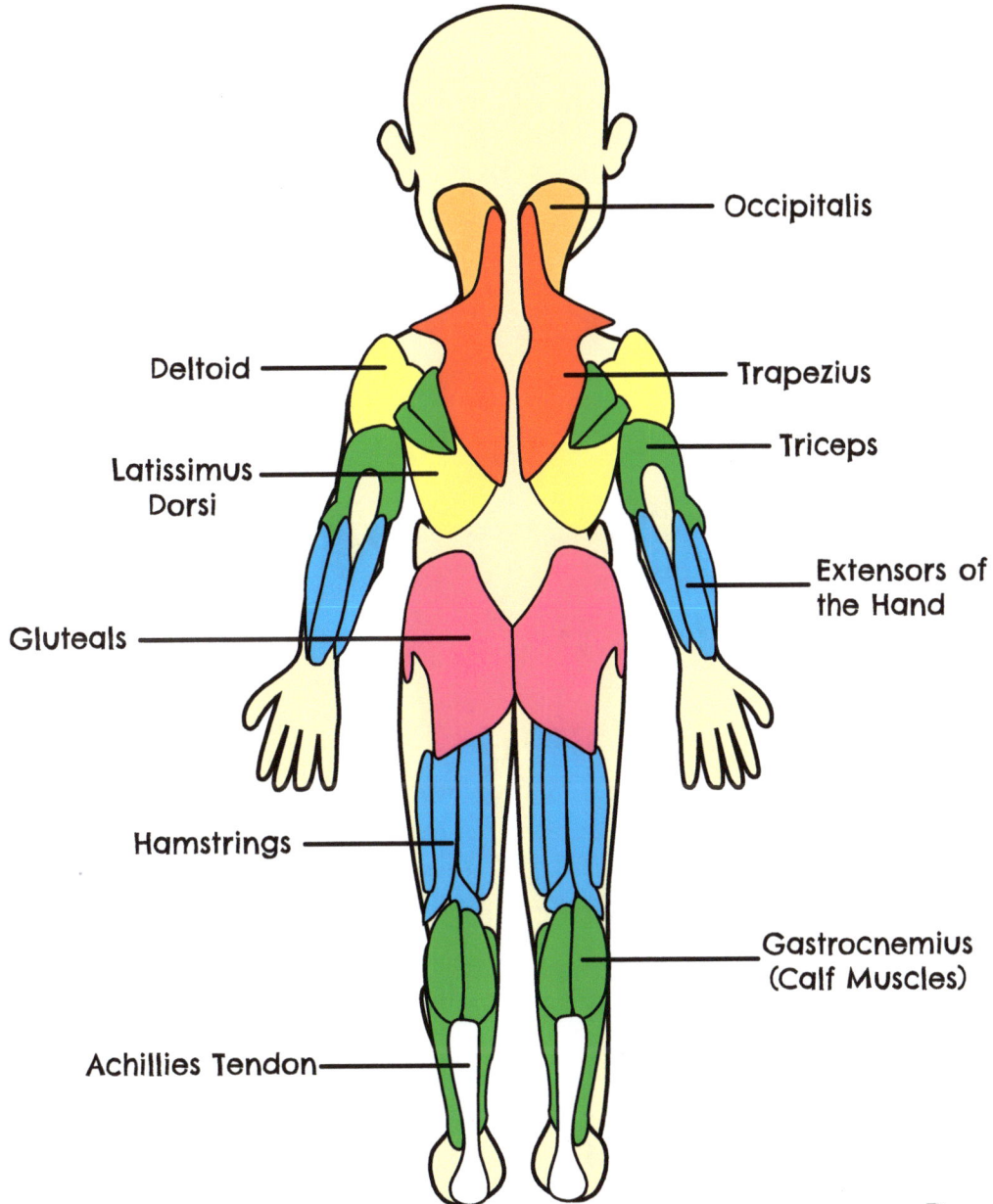

Occipitalis

Deltoid

Trapezius

Triceps

Latissimus
Dorsi

Extensors of
the Hand

Gluteals

Hamstrings

Gastrocnemius
(Calf Muscles)

Achillies Tendon

Dumbbell Bicep Curls

Hold a dumbbell in each hand
Stand with your feet as wide as your hips
Let your arms hang down at your sides
Stand tall with your body
Keep your knees a little bent
Curl both arms up to meet your shoulders
Slowly lower the dumbbells back down
Can you do this 5 times?

1.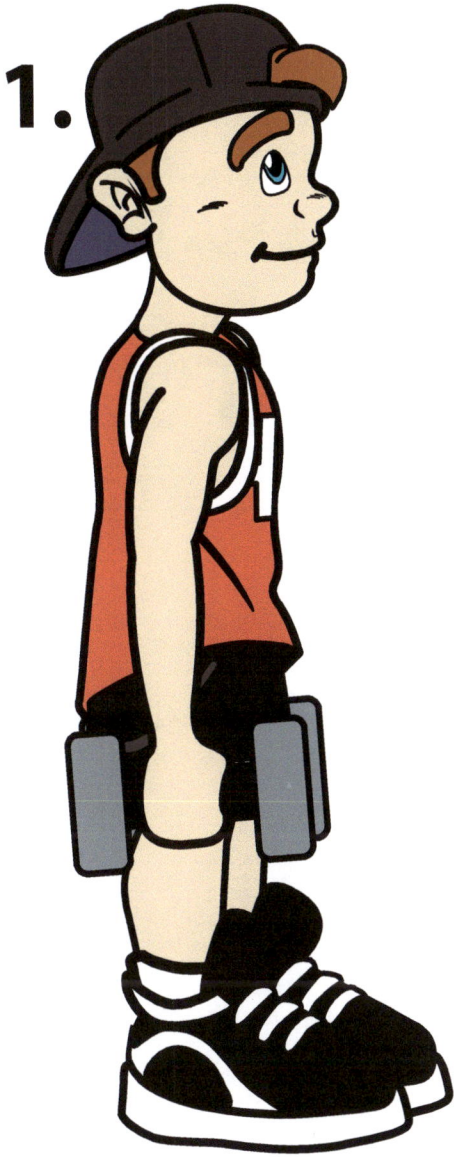

2.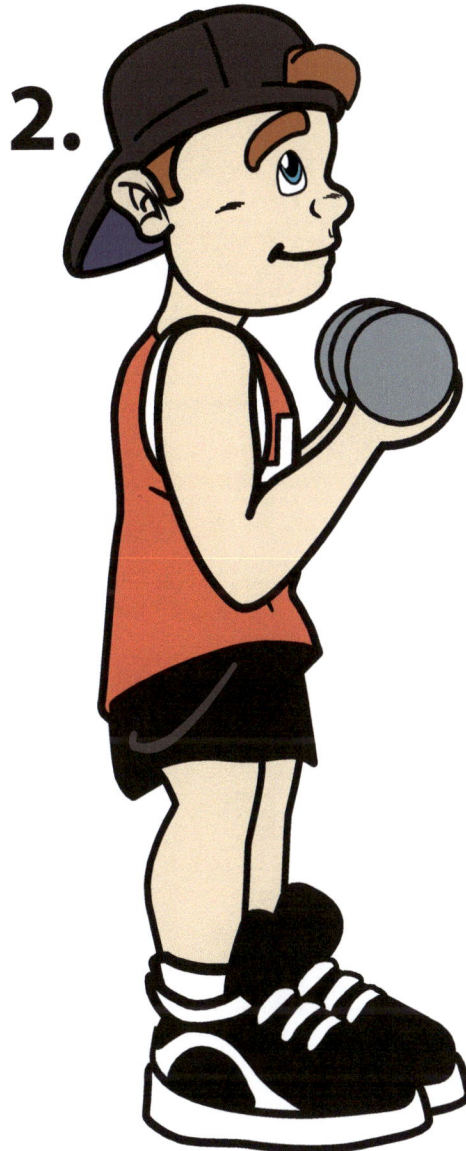

Dumbbell Tricep Kick Backs

Hold a dumbbell in each hand

Keep your upper arms by your sides

Lift the dumbbells until your arms

are back and straight

Slowly lower the dumbbells back down

Can you do this 5 times?

1.

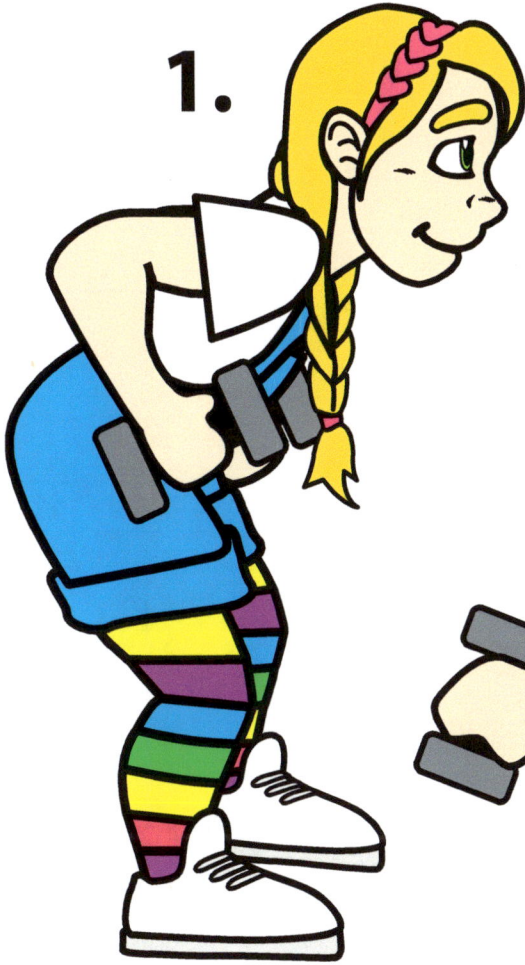

2.

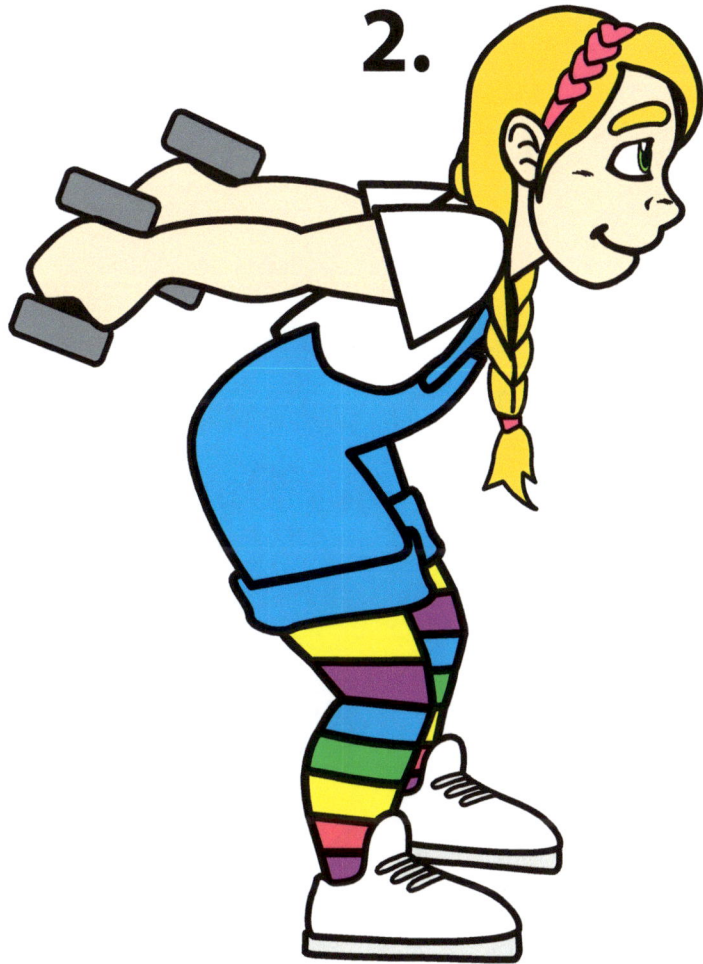

Dumbbell Lying Chest Press

Lie on the floor with a dumbbell in each hand
Bend your knees with your feet flat on the floor
Push the dumbbells up so your arms
are in line over your shoulders
Touch the dumbbells together
Lower the dumbbells down until your
elbows touch the floor
Can you do this 5 times?

1.

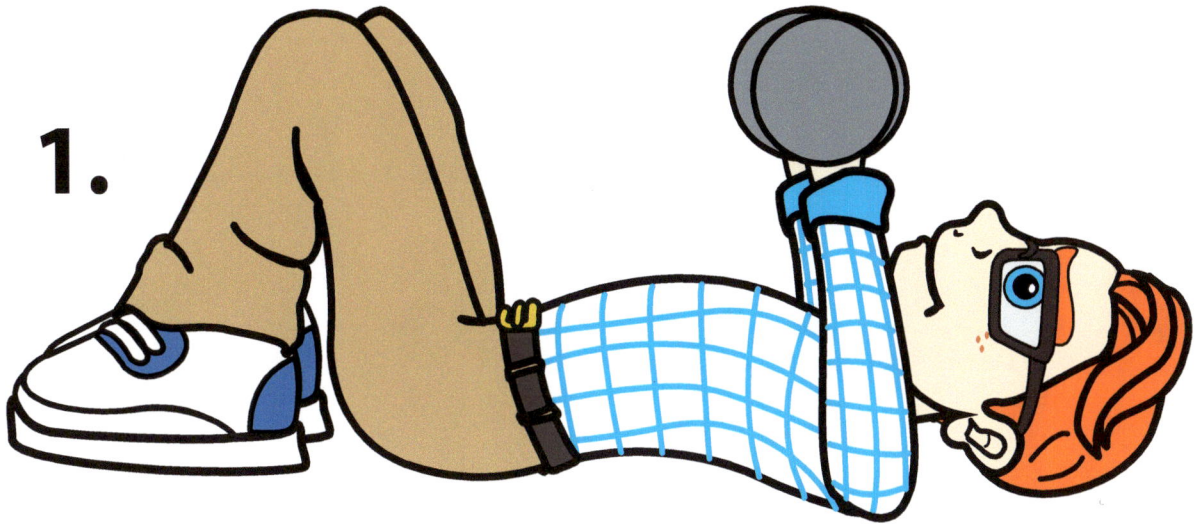

2.

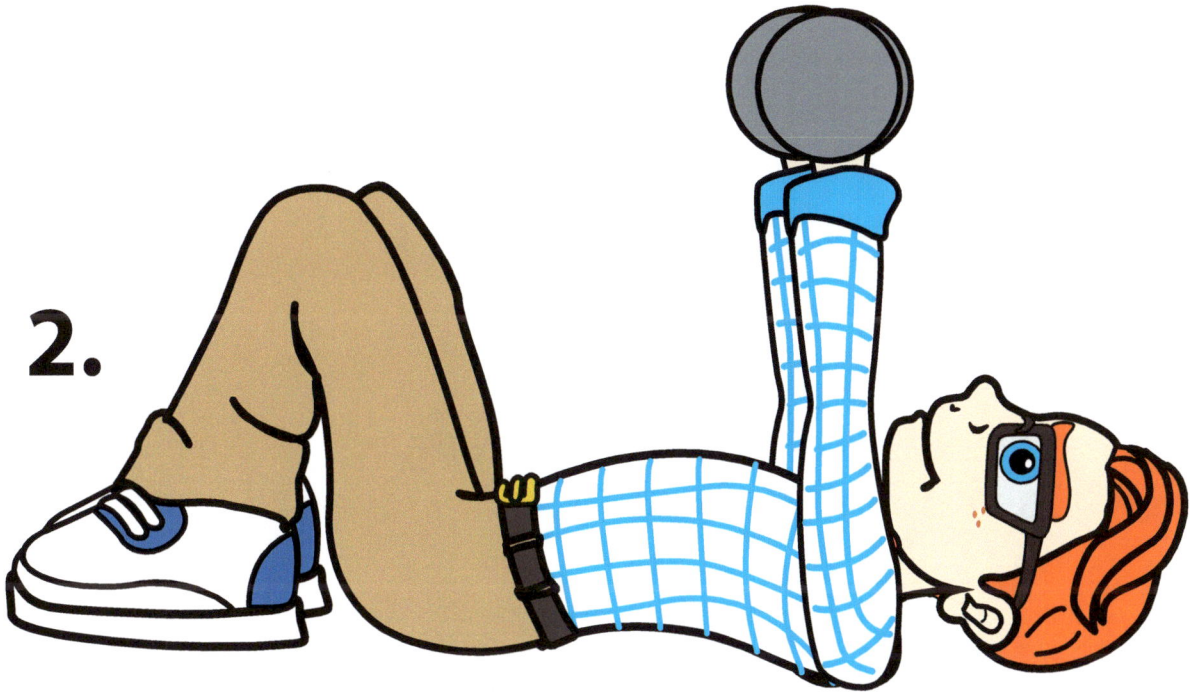

Dumbbell Lateral Raises

Stand up tall with your legs as wide
as your shoulders

Hold a dumbbell in each hand beside you

Lift the dumbbells up to your shoulders

Keep your elbows a little bent

Slowly lower the dumbbells back to the start

Can you do this 5 times?

1.

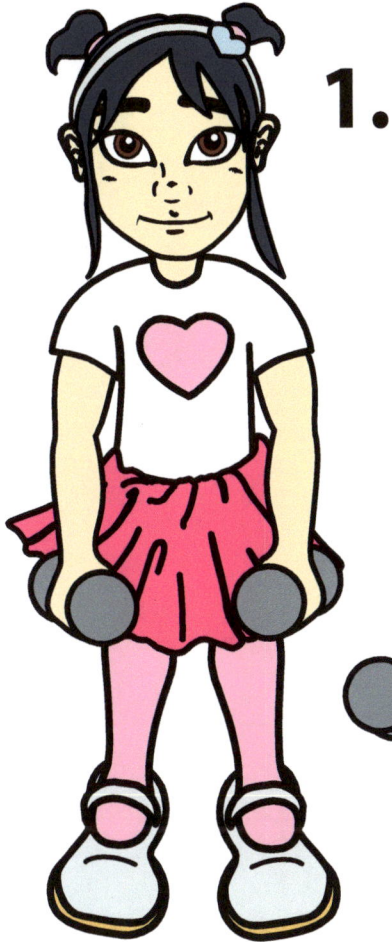

2.

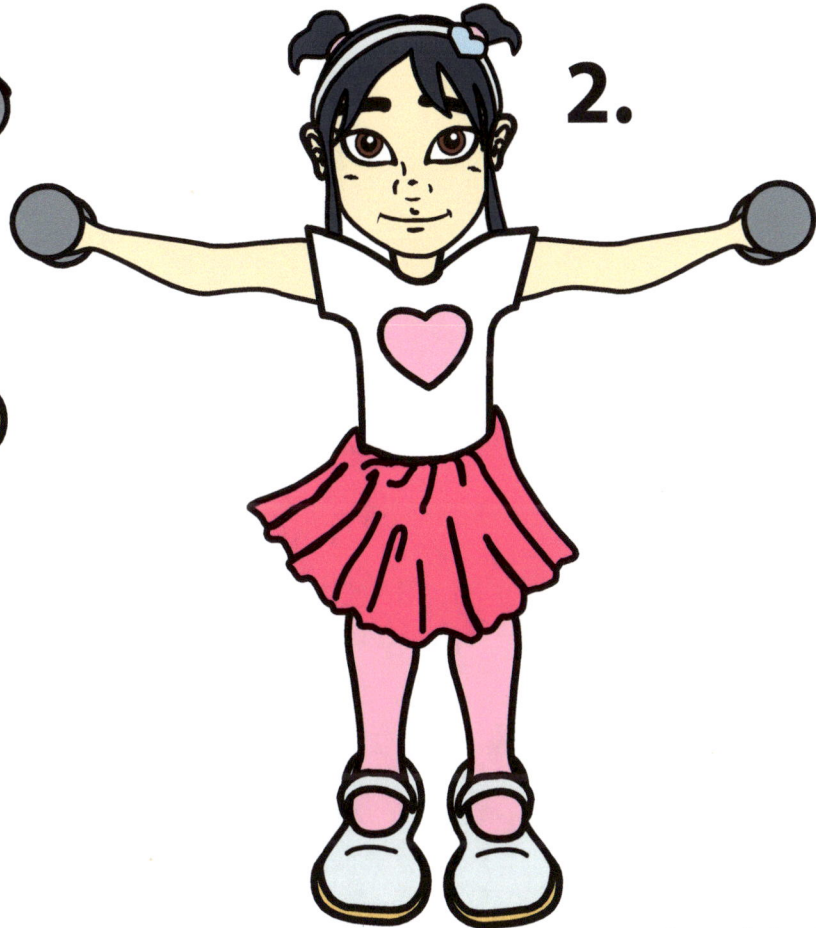

Dumbbells 13

Dumbbell Lunges

Stand up tall with a dumbbell in
each hand by your sides
Step forward with your right leg
Keep your body straight while you lower
your upper body down
Keep that balance and return back
to standing position
Can you do this 5 times?

1.

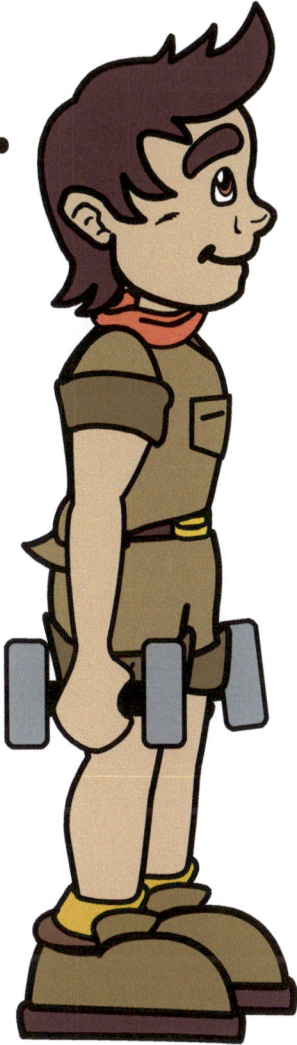

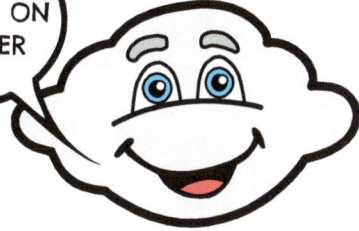

2.

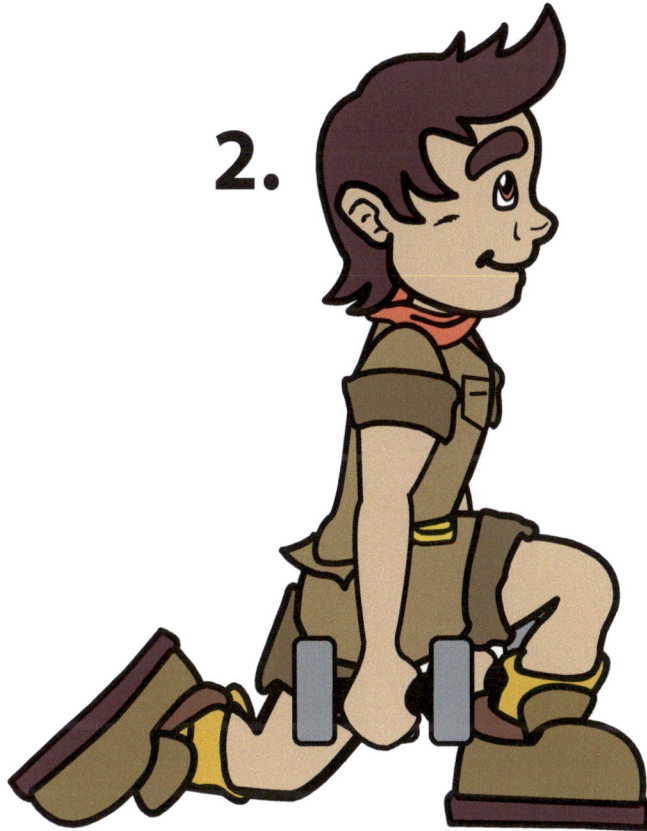

Dumbbell Upright Rows

Hold a dumbbell in each hand

Stand with your legs as wide as your shoulders

Slowly use your shoulders to lift
the dumbbells up

Keep the dumbbells close to your body as you lift

Use your elbows to lift the dumbbells up

Slowly lower them down

Can you do this 5 times?

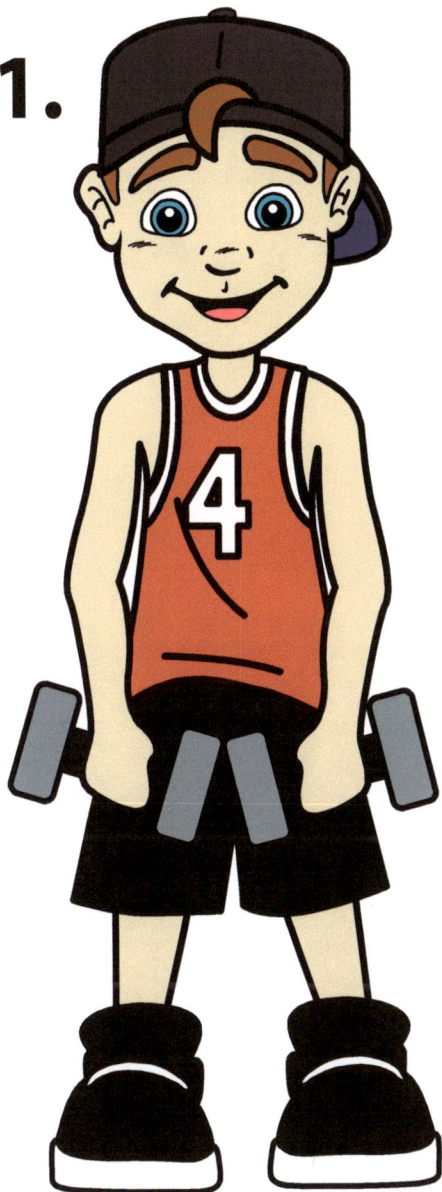

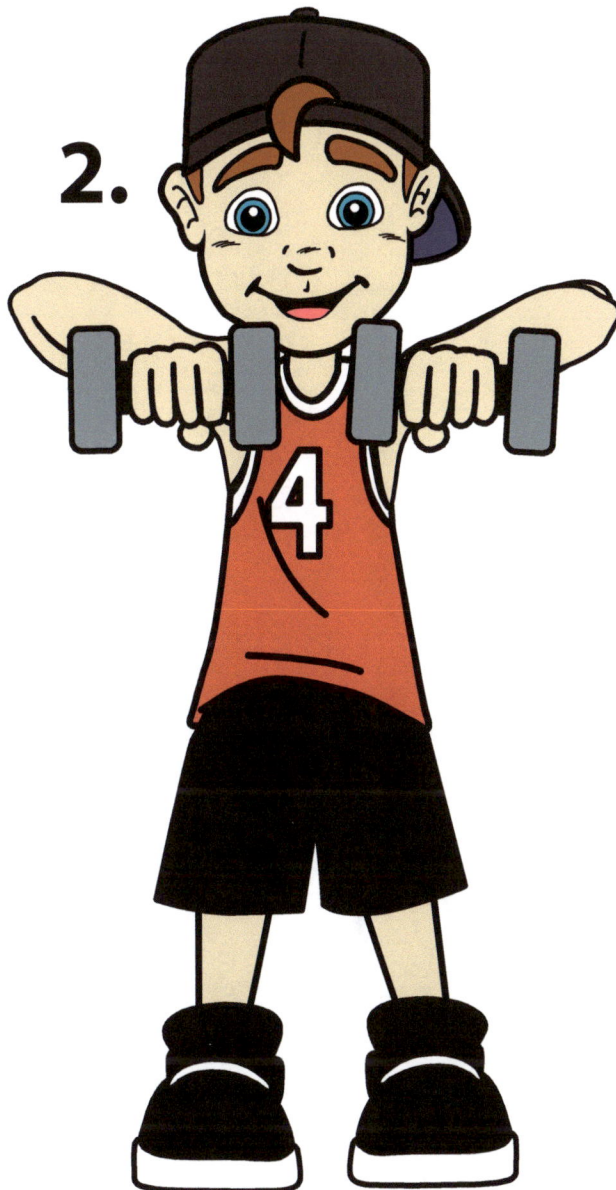

1.

2.

Dumbbells 17

Dumbbell Bent Over Rows

Bend your upper body forward
Hold a dumbbell in each hand in
front of your body
Keep your back straight
Slowly lift the dumbbells to your side
Keep your elbows close to your body
Slowly lower the dumbbells back to the start
Can you do this 5 times?

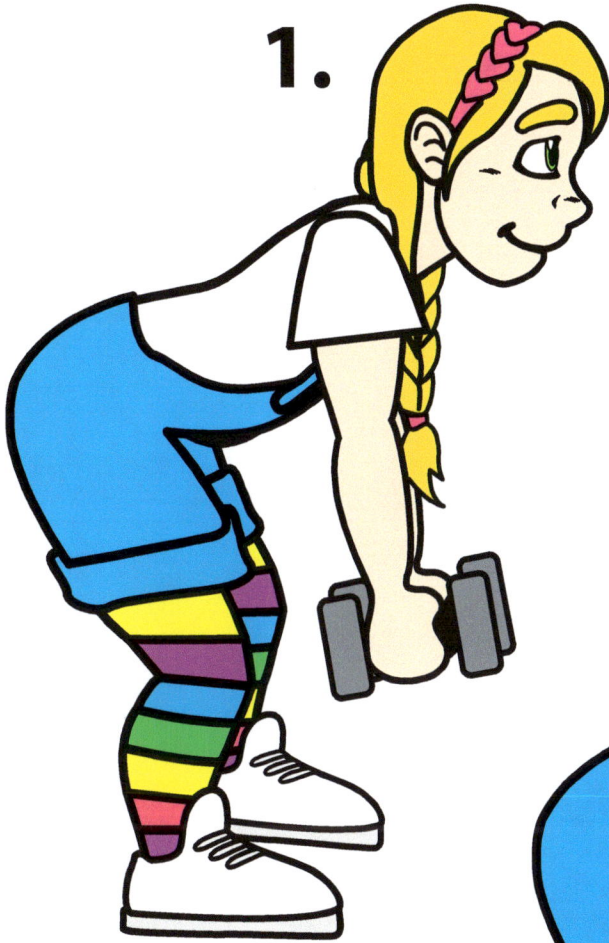

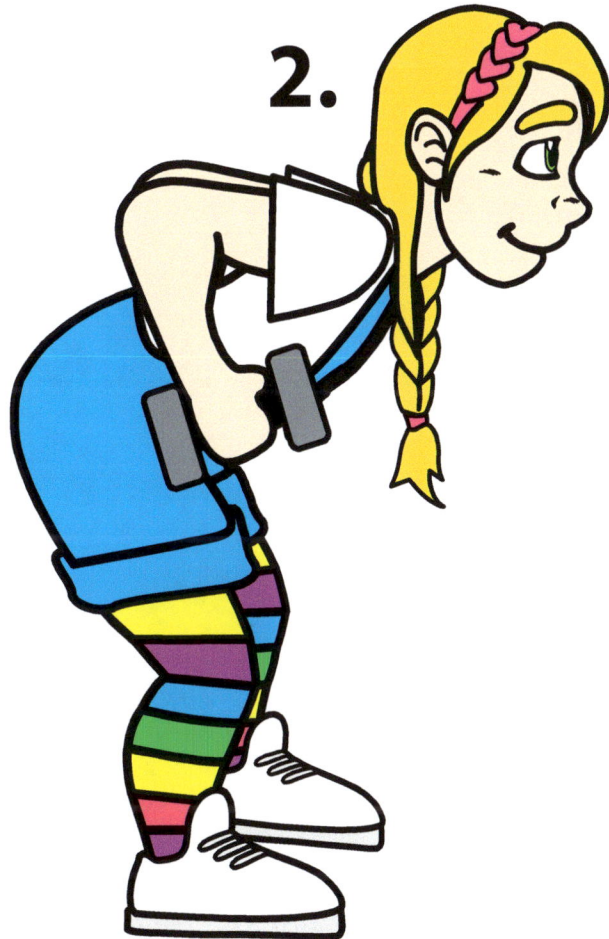

Dumbbell Shoulder Press

Hold a dumbbell in each hand in
line with your shoulders
Keep your chest up and your core
tight Push the dumbbells up until
your arms are straight
Touch the weights above your head.
Slowly lower the dumbbells back down
Can you do this 5 times?

1.

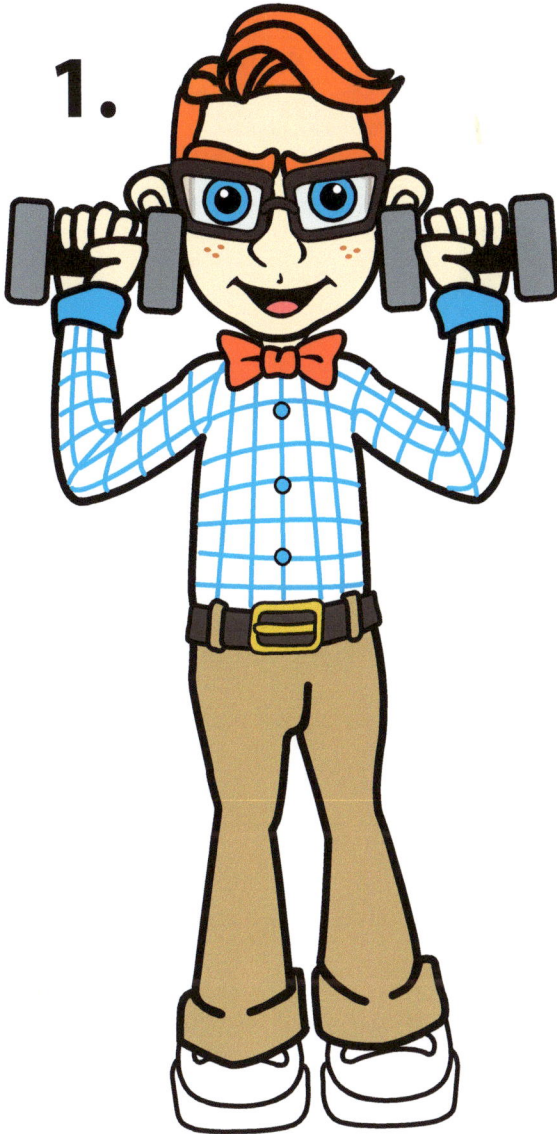

2.

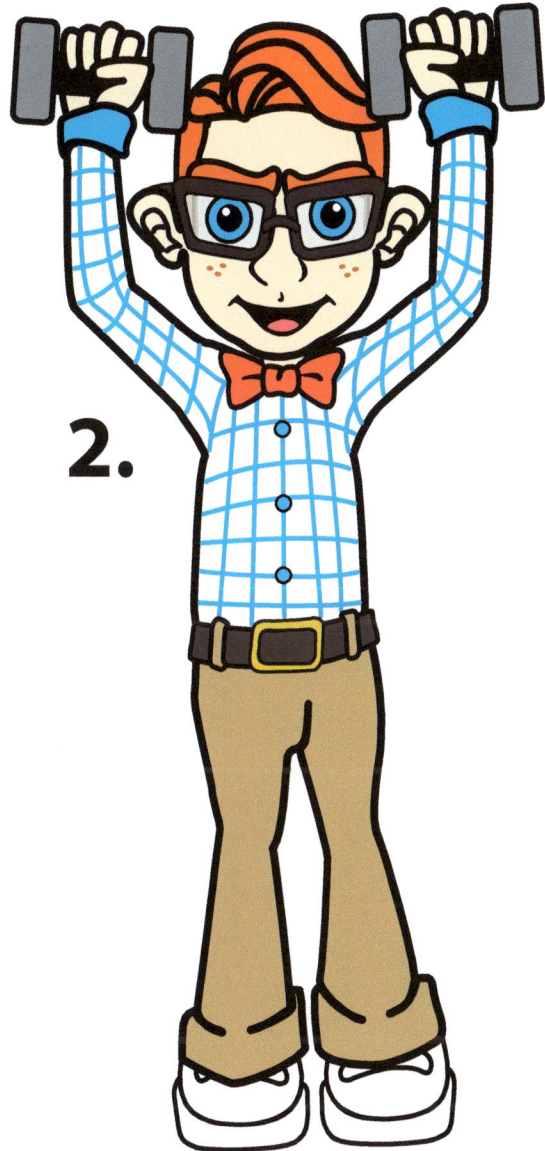

Dumbbell Sumo Squats

Stand tall with your feet apart
Stand with your legs as wide as your shoulders
Turn your toes slightly out
Hold the dumbbells with both hands
Hold them near your chest together
Lower your body back as far as you can
Push your hips back
Bend your knees
Slowly stand back up again
Can you do this 5 times?

1.

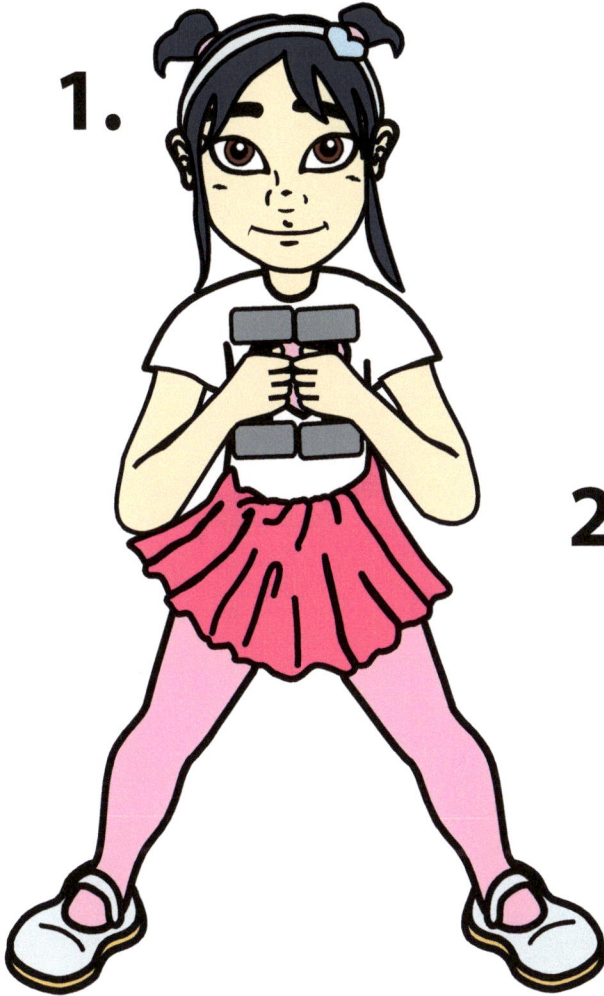

2.

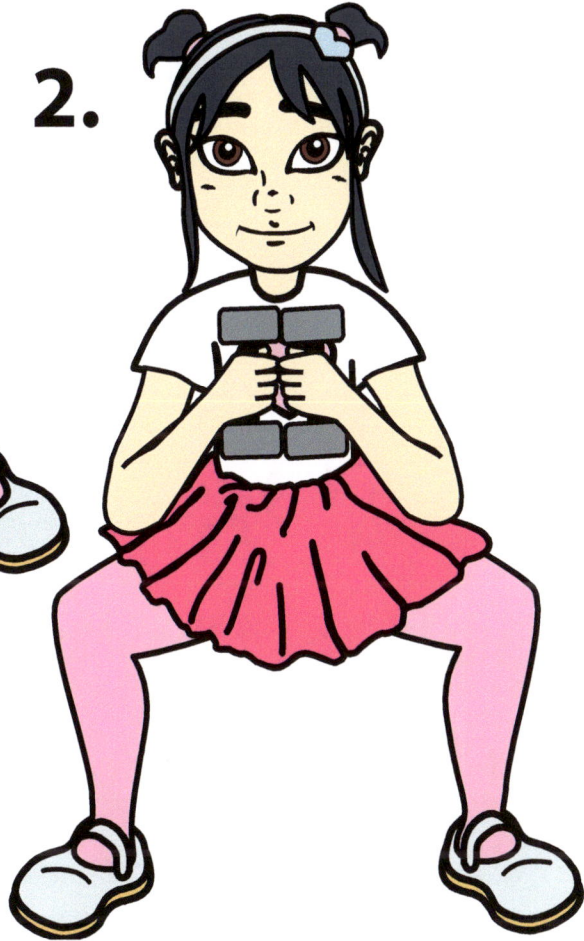

Dumbbell Deadlifts

Stand up tall with your legs as
wide as your shoulders
Hold a dumbbell in each hand in front of you
Bend your knees a little
Lower the dumbbells to the
top of your feet
Slowly bring the dumbbells back
up to starting position
Can you do this 5 times?

1.

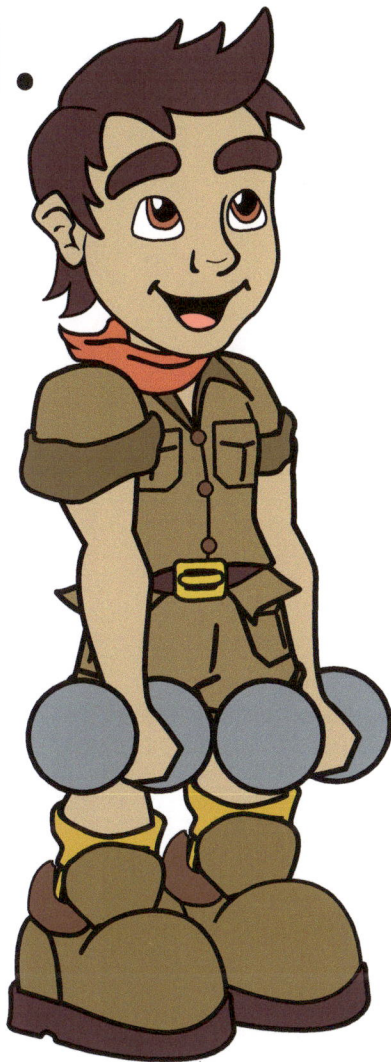

2.

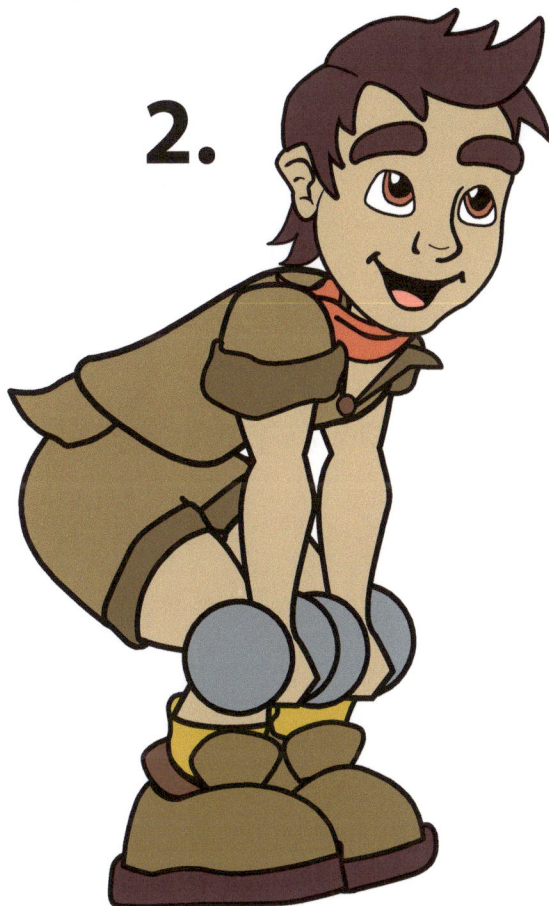

Dumbbell Lying Flyes

Lie on the floor on your back
Bend your knees with your feet flat on the floor
Lift the dumbbells so they are above
you in line with your chest
Face your palms to each other
Bend your elbows
Lower your arms in a wide arc
to open your chest
Bring your arms back up to the start
Can you do this 5 times?

1.

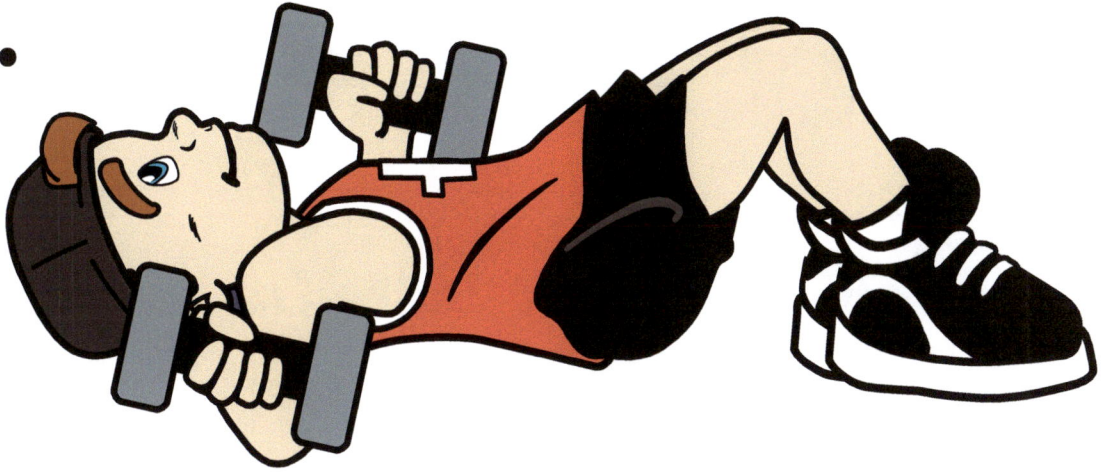

2.

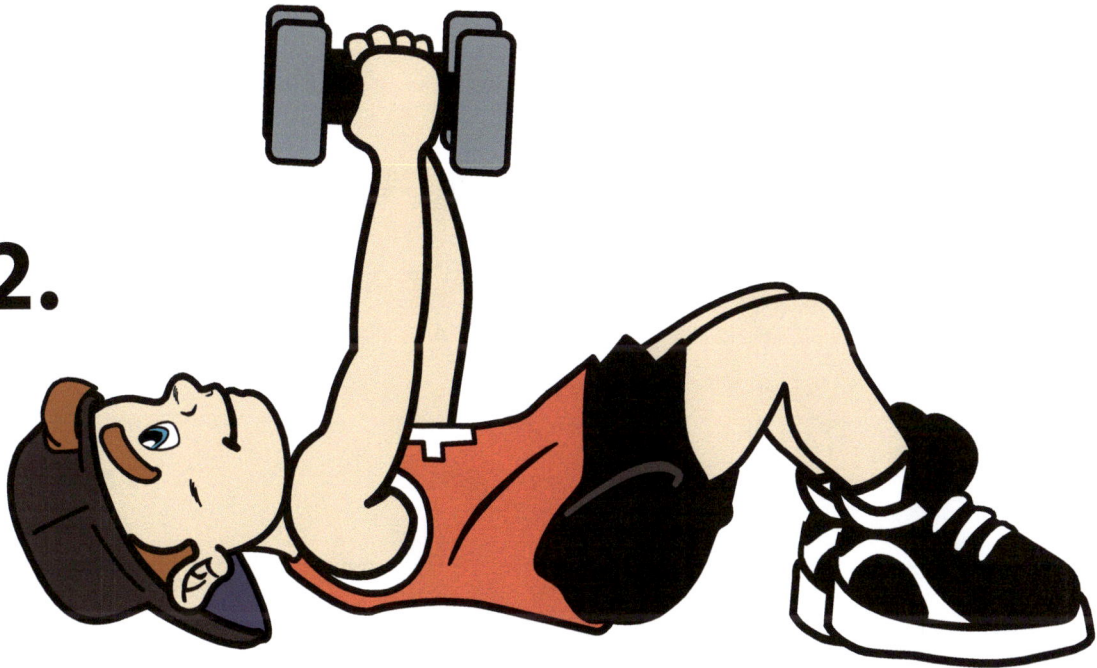

Dumbbell Crunches

Lie on the floor on your back

Bend your knees with your feet flat on the floor

Hold a dumbbell with two hands

Hold your arms straight above your shoulders

Slowly lift your upper body up and

squeeze your stomach

Lower your body back down

slowly to the floor

Can you do this 5 times?

1.

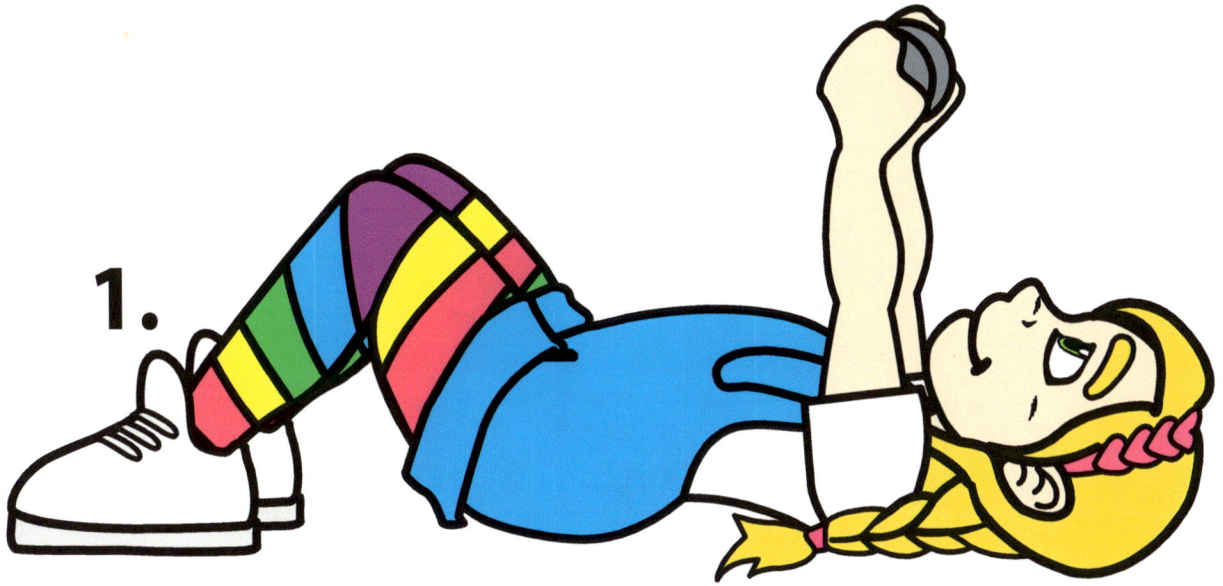

2.

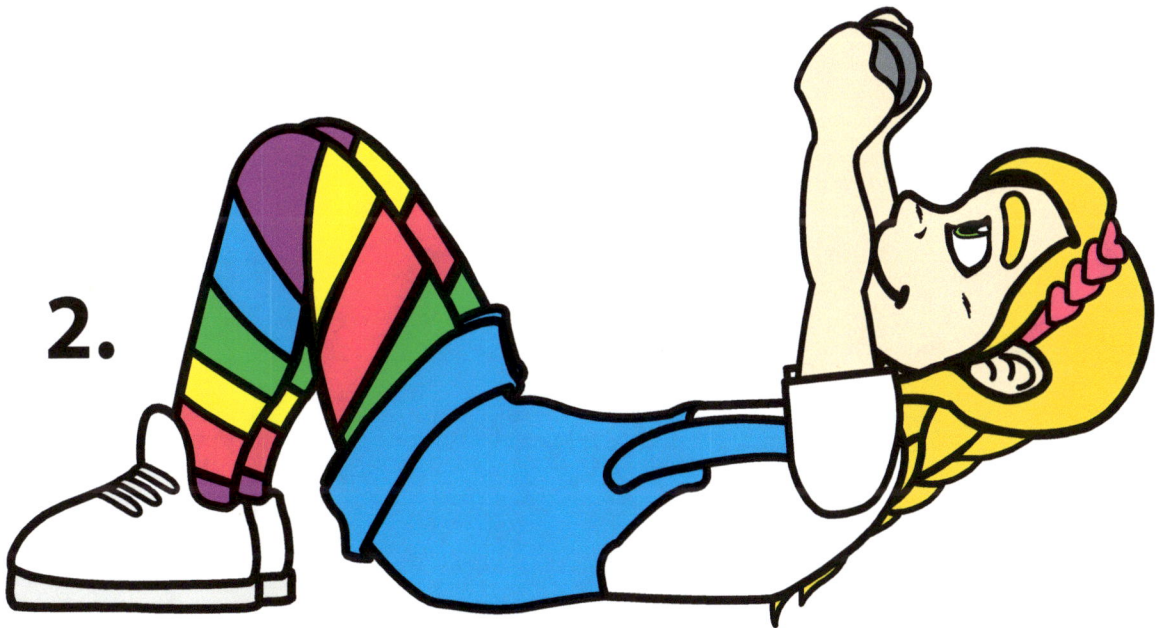

Dumbbell Arm Circles

Stand up straight

Place your feet as wide as your shoulders

Hold a dumbbell in each hand

Lift your arms straight out by your sides

Slowly make circles with your
arms moving forward

Repeat this action going backwards

Can you do this 5 times each way?

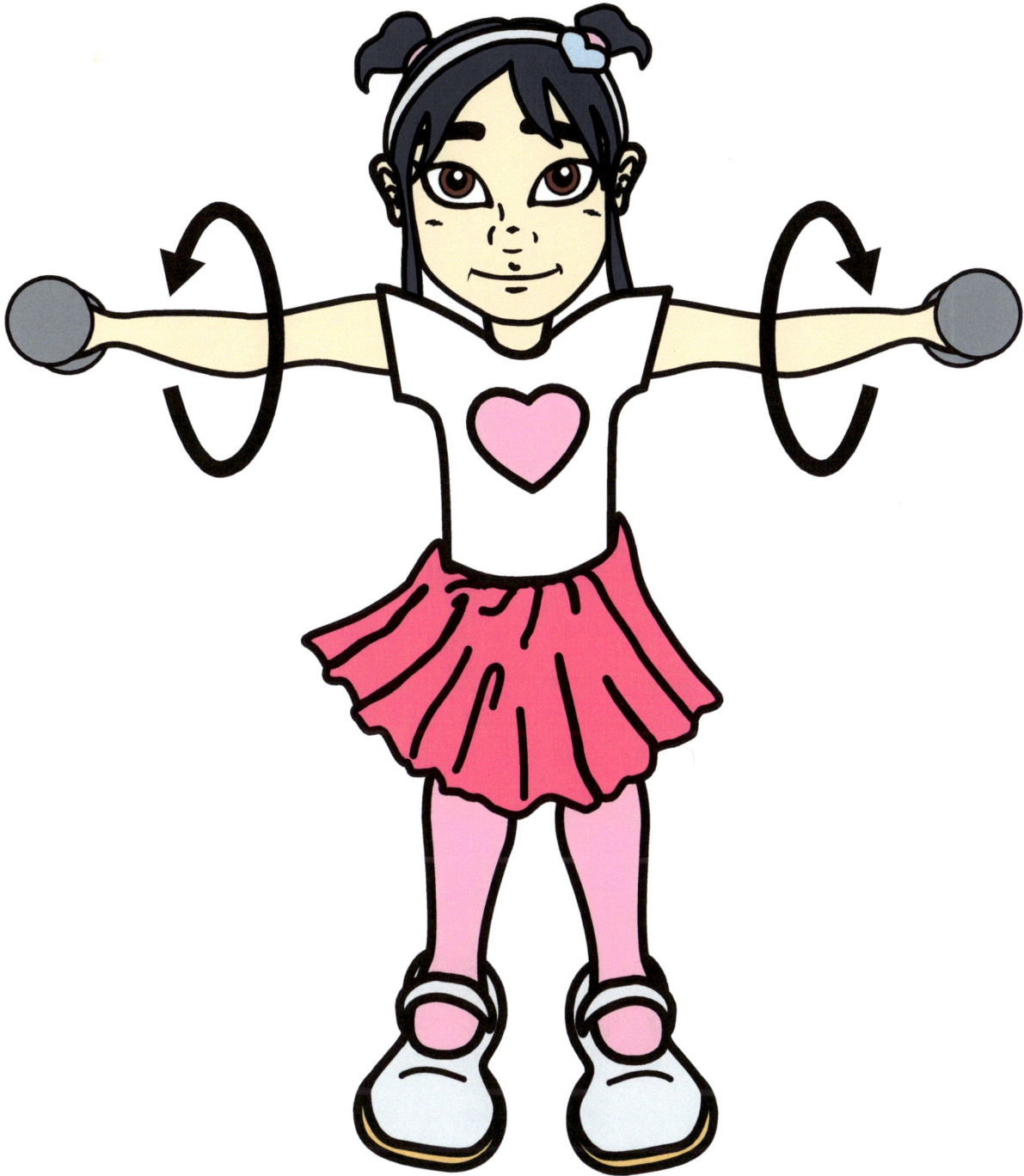

Dumbbell Calf Raises

Stand up tall with your legs as wide
as your shoulders

Hold a dumbbell in each hand beside you

Raise your heels off the floor

Hold your balance at the top

Slowly lower your heels back to the floor

Can you do this 5 times?

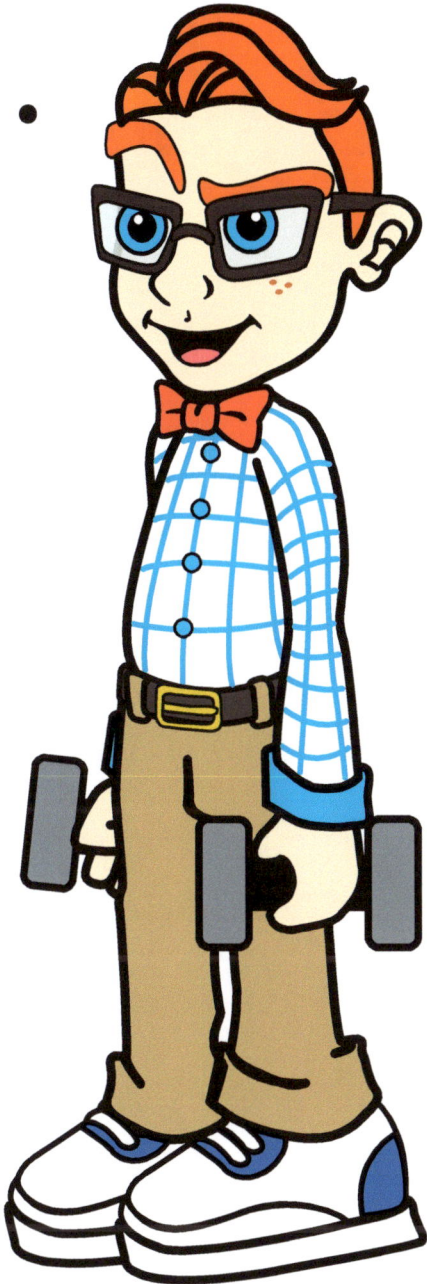

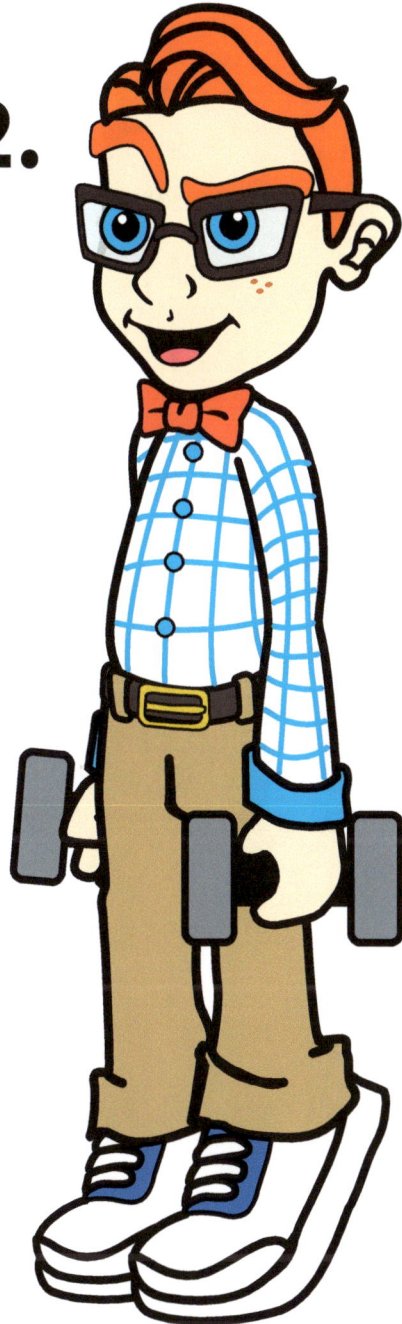

1.

2.

Dumbbell Squats

Stand up tall with a dumbbell in each hand

Face your toes slightly out

Slowly bend the knees and lower your legs

Keep your back straight

Bend down only until your hip is in

line with your knees

Slowly stand back up

Can you do this 5 times?

1.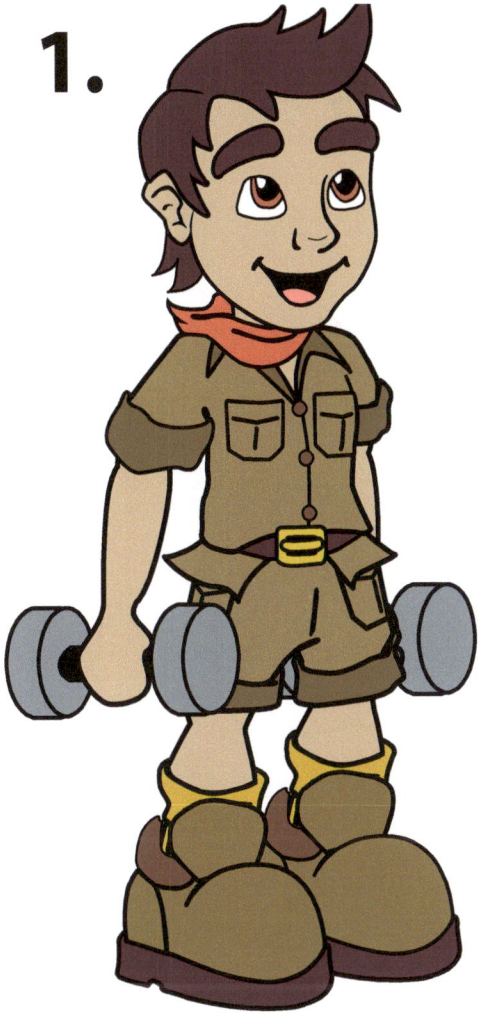

2.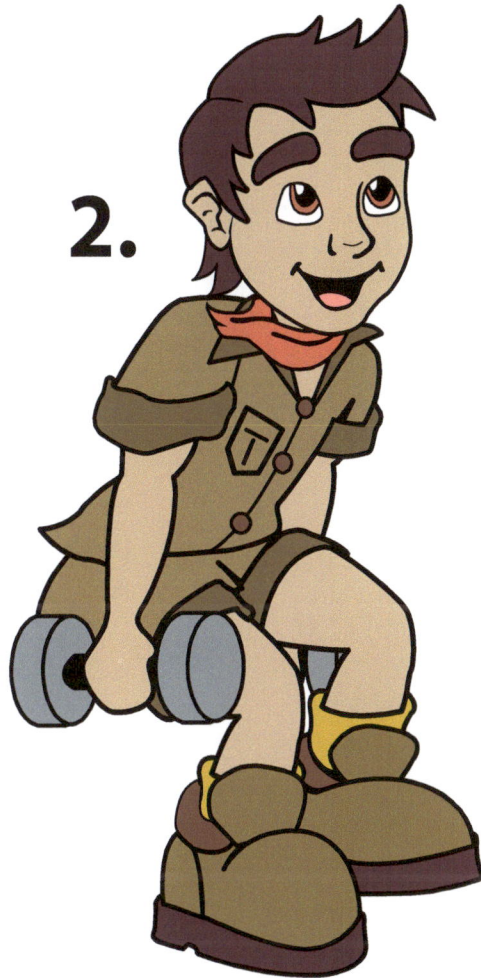

Keep an eye out for the rest of the series

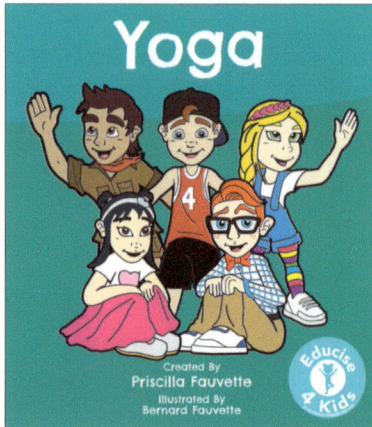

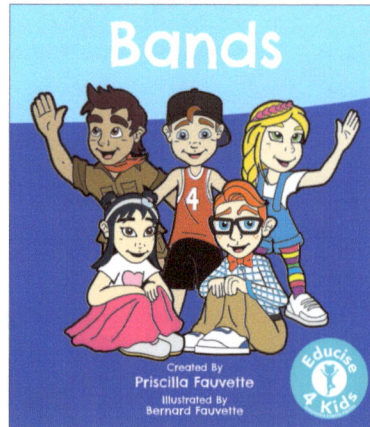

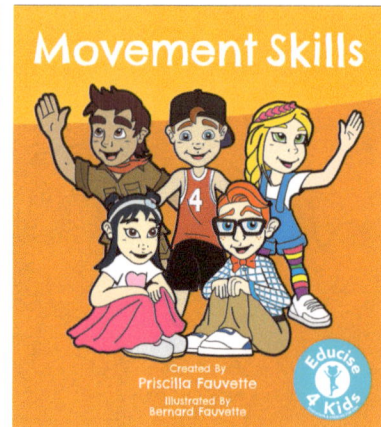

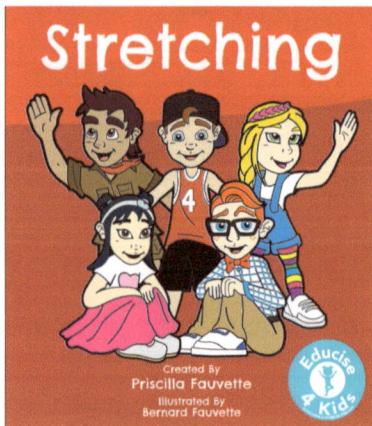

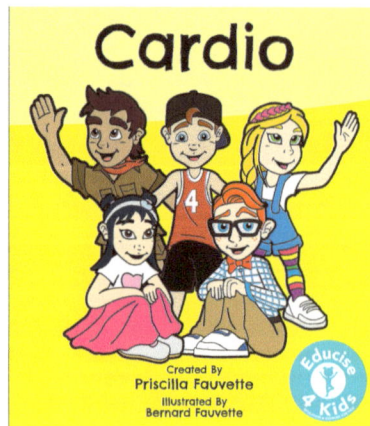

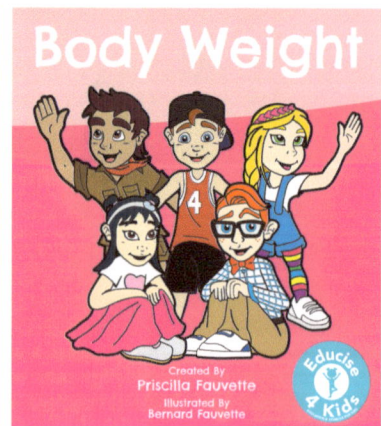

Yoga
Created By Priscilla Fauvette
Illustrated By Bernard Fauvette
Educise 4 Kids

Bands
Created By Priscilla Fauvette
Illustrated By Bernard Fauvette
Educise 4 Kids

Movement Skills
Created By Priscilla Fauvette
Illustrated By Bernard Fauvette
Educise 4 Kids

Stretching
Created By Priscilla Fauvette
Illustrated By Bernard Fauvette
Educise 4 Kids

Cardio
Created By Priscilla Fauvette
Illustrated By Bernard Fauvette
Educise 4 Kids

Body Weight
Created By Priscilla Fauvette
Illustrated By Bernard Fauvette
Educise 4 Kids

www.ingramcontent.com/pod-product-compliance
Lightning Source LLC
Chambersburg PA
CBHW061137030426
42334CB00003B/78